I0697079

Holistic Health Guide Made Easy for Beginners

Developing Your Holistic Health Plan

By

Emory Lasse

Copyright@2023

Table of Contents

CHAPTER 1

Introduction

Holistic health is a comprehensive and integrative approach to well-being that considers the whole person - mind, body, emotions, and spirit - rather than focusing solely on specific symptoms or diseases. It recognizes that all aspects of an individual's life are interconnected and influence their overall health and wellness. This holistic perspective emphasizes the importance of achieving balance and harmony within these various dimensions to attain optimal health.

1.1 What Is Holistic Health

At its core, holistic health seeks to understand health and illness within the broader context of a person's life. It goes beyond just treating physical symptoms and acknowledges the interplay between physical, mental, emotional, and spiritual health. Here are some key components of holistic health:

- **Physical Health:** This aspect involves maintaining the body's physical well-being through proper nutrition, regular exercise, and minimizing exposure to toxins and harmful substances. It also encompasses understanding how physical health can affect mental and emotional well-being.

- **Mental Health:** Holistic health recognizes the significance of mental health in overall well-being. It involves managing stress, fostering positive thought patterns, and nurturing cognitive health. Techniques such as mindfulness and meditation are often incorporated to support mental well-being.

- **Emotional Health:** Emotional health encompasses the ability to recognize, express, and manage one's emotions effectively. It involves cultivating emotional resilience, empathy, and healthy relationships. Emotions are seen as integral to the overall health picture.

- **Spiritual Health:** This dimension addresses questions of meaning, purpose, and connection to something greater than oneself. It doesn't necessarily involve religious beliefs but rather a sense of inner peace, purpose, and alignment with personal values.

- **Social Health:** Holistic health recognizes the importance of social connections and relationships. Maintaining healthy relationships and a support network is considered vital for overall well-being.

- **Environmental Health:** This aspect acknowledges the impact of the external environment on one's health. It involves making choices that promote a healthy environment, such as reducing exposure to pollution and toxins.

- **Holistic Therapies:** Holistic health often incorporates alternative therapies like acupuncture, herbal medicine, chiropractic care, and energy healing. These therapies aim to address imbalances in the body's energy or systems and promote natural healing.

1.2 Why Holistic Health Matters for Beginners

Holistic health matters, especially for beginners, because it offers a more holistic view of health and wellness that empowers individuals to take control of their well-being. Here's why it's essential for newcomers to the concept:

- **Comprehensive Understanding:** Holistic health provides a comprehensive understanding of health, recognizing that physical symptoms are often interconnected with mental, emotional, and spiritual factors. This broader perspective can lead to more effective and lasting solutions.

- **Preventive Approach:** It emphasizes preventive measures, helping individuals make healthier lifestyle choices that can prevent illness and promote long-term well-being.

- **Personal Empowerment:** Beginners in holistic health learn to take an active role in their health journey. They are encouraged to make informed choices and adopt practices that align with their unique needs and values.

- **Reduced Reliance on Medications:** For those seeking

alternatives or complementary approaches to conventional medicine, holistic health offers various natural and non-invasive therapies that can reduce reliance on medications and their potential side effects.

- **Enhanced Quality of Life:** Holistic health practices often lead to an improved quality of life. By addressing mental and emotional well-being alongside physical health, individuals can experience greater overall satisfaction and happiness.

1.3 Setting Your Holistic Health Goals

Setting holistic health goals is a pivotal step for beginners because it

provides a clear roadmap for their
health and well-being journey. Here's
how to approach this process:

- **Self-Assessment:** Begin by
  assessing your current state of
  health in all dimensions: physical,
  mental, emotional, spiritual, and
  social. Take stock of your
  strengths and areas that need
  improvement.

- **Identify Priorities:** Determine
  which aspects of holistic health are
  most important to you. Is it
  reducing stress, improving
  physical fitness, enhancing
  emotional resilience, or exploring
  spiritual practices?

- **SMART Goals:** Utilize the
  SMART (Specific, Measurable,
  Achievable, Relevant, Time-
  bound) criteria to set specific and

achievable goals. For example, instead of a vague goal like "be healthier," you might set a SMART goal like "exercise for 30 minutes, five days a week, for the next three months."

- **Break It Down:** Break larger goals into smaller, manageable steps. This makes the process less overwhelming and allows you to track your progress more effectively.

- **Seek Guidance:** Consider consulting with a holistic health practitioner or coach who can help you set appropriate goals based on your individual needs and provide guidance along the way.

- **Regular Evaluation:** Periodically assess your progress and adjust your goals as needed. Holistic health is an ongoing journey, and flexibility is essential.

The introduction to holistic health provides a foundational understanding of this holistic approach to well-being, highlighting its importance for beginners. Setting holistic health goals empowers individuals to take charge of their health journey and work towards a balanced and fulfilling life that encompasses all aspects of their being.

CHAPTER 2

Understanding the Mind-Body Connection

The mind-body connection is a fundamental concept in holistic health that emphasizes the intricate relationship between mental and physical health.

2.1 Exploring the Mind-Body Connection

The mind-body connection recognizes that our thoughts, emotions, and mental states can profoundly influence our physical well-being.

Here are some key points to consider in exploring this connection:

- **Neuroscience and Psychoneuroimmunology:** Scientific research has demonstrated that our thoughts and emotions can affect the nervous and immune systems. Positive emotions and thoughts can enhance immune function, while stress and negativity can weaken it.

- **The Power of the Placebo Effect:** The placebo effect showcases how belief and expectation can impact physical outcomes. It highlights the mind's ability to influence the body's response to treatment.

- **Stress and Health:** Chronic stress can lead to a range of physical health issues, including cardiovascular problems, digestive disorders, and weakened immunity. Understanding how to manage stress is crucial for overall well-being.

- **Mindful Awareness:** Mindfulness practices, such as meditation and deep breathing, can help individuals become more aware of their thoughts and emotions. This awareness is a key step in harnessing the mind-body connection for improved health.

2.2 How Emotions Impact Your Health

This subsection delves deeper into the role of emotions in shaping physical health:

- **Emotional Resilience:** Emotional resilience refers to the ability to cope with life's challenges and bounce back from adversity. It is closely linked to overall health and well-being.

- **Negative Emotions and Health:** Chronic negative emotions like anger, anxiety, and sadness can contribute to health problems. They may lead to inflammation, weaken the immune system, and increase the risk of chronic diseases.

- **Positive Emotions and Health:** Conversely, positive emotions like joy, gratitude, and love have been linked to improved physical health outcomes. They can boost the immune system, reduce inflammation, and enhance overall vitality.

- **Emotional Intelligence:**
  Developing emotional intelligence, which includes recognizing and managing one's own emotions as well as understanding and empathizing with the emotions of others, is essential for achieving emotional balance and better health.

2.3 Practices for Achieving Mind-Body Balance

Achieving mind-body balance involves adopting practices and strategies that promote harmony between mental and physical well-being. Here are some practices to consider:

- **Mindfulness Meditation:** Regular mindfulness meditation cultivates awareness of thoughts and emotions, reducing stress and promoting mental clarity.

- **Yoga:** Yoga combines physical postures, breath control, and meditation to promote flexibility, relaxation, and a sense of inner peace.

- **Breathing Exercises:** Deep breathing exercises help calm the nervous system, reduce stress, and enhance oxygenation of the body's tissues.

- **Biofeedback:** Biofeedback techniques provide real-time data on physiological processes such as heart rate and muscle tension, enabling individuals to gain control over these functions.

- **Counseling and Therapy:**
  Seeking the support of a therapist
  or counselor can help individuals
  explore and manage their emotions
  in a safe and constructive way.

- **Creative Expression:** Engaging in
  creative activities like art, music,
  or writing can be therapeutic,
  allowing individuals to express
  and process their emotions.

- **Healthy Lifestyle Choices:** Proper
  nutrition, regular exercise, and
  adequate sleep are foundational for
  maintaining a healthy mind-body
  balance.

Incorporating these practices into
your life can help you harness the
power of the mind-body connection,
manage emotions effectively, and
promote overall well-being.
Understanding this connection and

actively working towards balance is a
key step on the journey to holistic
health.

CHAPTER 3

Nutrition and Holistic Health

Nutrition plays a pivotal role in holistic health, as it directly affects the body's physical, mental, and emotional well-being.

3.1 The Role of Nutrition in Holistic Health

Nutrition is the foundation of holistic health, as it provides the body with the essential nutrients it needs to function optimally. Here's why nutrition is crucial in the context of holistic health:

- **Physical Health:** Nutrition supplies the body with the necessary vitamins, minerals, carbohydrates, proteins, and fats needed for energy, growth, and repair. A well-balanced diet supports overall physical health, including the immune system, digestive system, and cardiovascular health.

- **Mental Clarity:** Proper nutrition is linked to cognitive function and mental clarity. Nutrient-rich foods can enhance memory, concentration, and mental alertness, contributing to overall mental well-being.

- **Emotional Stability:** Nutrition can influence mood and emotional stability. Consuming a diet rich in whole foods can help regulate blood sugar levels and reduce mood swings and irritability.

- **Inflammation and Disease Prevention:** A diet high in anti-inflammatory foods, such as fruits, vegetables, and omega-3 fatty acids, can help reduce the risk of chronic diseases associated with inflammation, such as heart disease and arthritis.

- **Gut Health:** Nutrition is closely tied to gut health, which in turn impacts overall well-being. A healthy gut microbiome is essential for digestion, nutrient absorption, and even mental health.

3.2 Building a Balanced Holistic Diet

Building a balanced holistic diet involves making conscious choices about the foods you consume to promote overall health and well-being. Here are key principles to consider:

- **Whole, Unprocessed Foods:** Focus on whole foods in their natural state, such as fruits, vegetables, whole grains, lean proteins, nuts, and seeds. These foods are rich in nutrients and free from additives and preservatives.

- **Variety:** Aim to incorporate a wide variety of foods to ensure you receive a broad spectrum of nutrients. Eating a rainbow of fruits and vegetables is a good practice.

- **Mindful Eating:** Pay attention to hunger and fullness cues, and eat slowly and attentively. This practice can help prevent overeating and promote digestion.

- **Hydration:** Proper hydration is essential for holistic health. Drink plenty of water throughout the day to support bodily functions.

- **Balanced Macronutrients:** Include a balance of carbohydrates, proteins, and healthy fats in your diet. These macronutrients provide energy and support various bodily functions.

- **Limit Processed Foods:** Minimize the consumption of highly processed and sugary foods, as they can lead to energy fluctuations and negatively affect overall health.

- **Listen to Your Body:** Be attuned to your body's unique needs and make dietary choices that align with your individual health goals and sensitivities.

- **Herbs and Supplements:** Consider incorporating herbs and supplements that support your specific health needs, but consult with a healthcare professional before adding them to your diet.

- **Food Sensitivities:** Be aware of any food sensitivities or allergies you may have and avoid foods that trigger adverse reactions.

- **Holistic Approaches to Eating:** Consider holistic approaches to eating, such as intuitive eating, which promotes a healthy relationship with food and body image.

- **Local and Seasonal Foods:** Whenever possible, choose locally sourced and seasonal foods, as they may be fresher and more nutrient-dense.

- **Cultural and Ethical Considerations:** Take into account your cultural and ethical values when making food choices, and explore ways to align your diet with these values.

Building a balanced holistic diet is not just about what you eat but also how you eat. It involves mindful choices, an understanding of the connection between nutrition and well-being, and a commitment to nourishing your body in a way that supports holistic health. This section empowers beginners to make informed choices about their dietary habits to enhance their overall wellness.

3.3 Superfoods and Supplements for Beginners

Superfoods and supplements can be valuable additions to a holistic diet, providing essential nutrients and health benefits.

Superfoods for Beginners:

1. **Berries:** Berries like blueberries, strawberries, and acai berries are rich in antioxidants, vitamins, and fiber. They can support cognitive function and boost the immune system.

2. **Leafy Greens:** Leafy greens such as kale, spinach, and Swiss chard are nutrient powerhouses, providing vitamins, minerals, and phytonutrients. They promote

overall health and may reduce the risk of chronic diseases.

3. **Nuts and Seeds:** Almonds, walnuts, chia seeds, and flaxseeds are high in healthy fats, protein, and fiber. They can support heart health, brain function, and digestion.

4. **Turmeric:** Turmeric contains curcumin, a potent anti-inflammatory compound. It can help reduce inflammation in the body and support joint health.

5. **Fatty Fish:** Fatty fish like salmon, mackerel, and sardines are rich in omega-3 fatty acids, which are beneficial for heart and brain health.

6. **Green Tea:** Green tea is loaded with antioxidants and may boost metabolism, aid in weight

management, and support overall well-being.

7. **Avocado:** Avocado is a source of healthy fats, fiber, and various vitamins and minerals. It supports skin health, digestion, and satiety.

8. **Probiotic Foods:** Fermented foods like yogurt, kefir, and sauerkraut contain beneficial probiotics that promote gut health and enhance digestion.

9. **Legumes:** Beans, lentils, and chickpeas are rich in fiber, protein, and various nutrients. They can help regulate blood sugar and support digestive health.

10. **Dark Chocolate:** Dark chocolate with a high cocoa content contains antioxidants and may have mood-boosting and cardiovascular

benefits when consumed in moderation.

Supplements for Beginners:

Before incorporating supplements into your holistic health regimen, it's essential to consult with a healthcare provider or registered dietitian to determine your specific needs. Here are some common supplements for beginners to consider:

1. **Multivitamins:** A high-quality multivitamin can provide essential vitamins and minerals that may be lacking in your diet.

2. **Vitamin D:** Vitamin D is crucial for bone health, immune function, and mood regulation. Many people have insufficient levels, especially if they have limited sun exposure.

3. **Omega-3 Fatty Acids:** Omega-3 supplements, such as fish oil or algae oil capsules, can support heart and brain health.

4. **Probiotics:** Probiotic supplements can help maintain a healthy gut microbiome, especially if you have digestive issues or have taken antibiotics recently.

5. **Vitamin B12:** If you follow a vegetarian or vegan diet, vitamin B12 supplementation may be necessary, as it is primarily found in animal products.

6. **Iron:** Iron supplements may be needed if you have a diagnosed iron deficiency or are at risk of developing one.

7. **Magnesium:** Magnesium supplements can support muscle

function, relaxation, and overall well-being.

8. **Calcium:** If you have low dietary calcium intake or are at risk of osteoporosis, calcium supplements may be recommended.

9. **Turmeric (Curcumin) Supplements:** For those seeking the anti-inflammatory benefits of turmeric, curcumin supplements may provide a concentrated dose.

10. **Collagen:** Collagen supplements are popular for supporting skin, joint, and bone health. However, their efficacy varies, so choose reputable brands.

Supplements should complement a balanced diet, not replace it. It's essential to prioritize whole, nutrient-dense foods as the primary source of nutrients and use supplements to fill

in specific gaps or address specific
health concerns. Additionally,
working with a healthcare provider or
registered dietitian can help determine
which supplements, if any, are
suitable for your individual needs.

CHAPTER 4
Physical Well-Being

Physical well-being is a crucial aspect of holistic health, encompassing various factors that contribute to overall physical fitness and vitality.

4.1 Exercise and Its Importance

Exercise is a cornerstone of physical well-being and holistic health. It offers a wide range of benefits that extend beyond physical fitness:

- **Physical Fitness:** Regular exercise improves cardiovascular health, builds muscle strength, enhances flexibility, and helps maintain a healthy weight.

- **Mental Health:** Exercise releases endorphins, which are natural mood elevators. It can reduce stress, anxiety, and symptoms of depression.

- **Cognitive Function:** Physical activity supports cognitive function and may improve memory, concentration, and creativity.

- **Energy Levels:** Engaging in regular physical activity can increase overall energy levels and combat feelings of fatigue.

- **Sleep Quality:** Exercise can improve sleep quality, helping individuals fall asleep faster and enjoy deeper, more restorative sleep.

- **Immune Function:** Moderate exercise is associated with a strengthened immune system, reducing the risk of illness.

- **Social Connection:** Participating in group fitness classes or team sports can foster social connections and support emotional well-being.

- **Longevity:** Studies show that regular exercise is linked to a longer, healthier life.

4.2 Holistic Fitness Practices

Holistic fitness practices prioritize overall well-being and consider the interconnectedness of physical, mental, and emotional health. Here are some holistic fitness practices to explore:

- **Yoga:** Yoga combines physical postures, breath control, and meditation to promote flexibility, balance, and mental clarity. It's known for its holistic approach to fitness and well-being.

- **Pilates:** Pilates focuses on core strength, flexibility, and body awareness. It can improve posture, balance, and overall body function.

- **Tai Chi:** Tai Chi is a gentle, low-impact exercise that incorporates slow, flowing movements and deep breathing. It promotes relaxation, balance, and mental focus.

- **Functional Training:** Functional training emphasizes movements that mimic daily activities, improving overall functional fitness and reducing the risk of injury.

- **Outdoor Activities:** Activities like hiking, cycling, and outdoor sports not only provide physical fitness but also connect individuals with nature, promoting mental well-being.

- **Dance:** Dancing is a fun way to stay active while improving coordination, rhythm, and self-expression. Various dance styles cater to different fitness levels and preferences.

- **Martial Arts:** Martial arts disciplines like karate or Brazilian jiu-jitsu offer physical fitness, discipline, and stress relief.

- **Mindful Movement:** Practices like Feldenkrais and Alexander

Technique focus on body awareness, posture, and efficient movement patterns.

4.3 Managing Pain and Discomfort Holistically

Managing pain and discomfort holistically involves addressing physical discomfort without relying solely on medications or invasive treatments. Here are some holistic approaches:

- **Acupuncture:** Acupuncture involves the insertion of fine needles at specific points on the body to promote pain relief and balance energy flow.

- **Chiropractic Care:** Chiropractors use manual adjustments to the spine and joints to alleviate pain,

improve mobility, and support
overall well-being.

- **Physical Therapy:** Physical
  therapists employ exercises,
  stretches, and manual techniques
  to manage pain and improve
  physical function.

- **Massage Therapy:** Massage can
  help relieve muscle tension, reduce
  pain, and promote relaxation.
  Various techniques cater to
  different needs.

- **Mind-Body Techniques:**
  Mindfulness meditation, deep
  breathing exercises, and
  progressive muscle relaxation can
  help manage pain by reducing
  stress and promoting relaxation.

- **Herbal Remedies:** Some herbs
  and supplements, such as turmeric,
  ginger, and arnica, have anti-

inflammatory and pain-relieving properties. Consult with a healthcare professional before using them.

- **Diet and Nutrition:** An anti-inflammatory diet rich in fruits, vegetables, omega-3 fatty acids, and antioxidants can help manage chronic pain and support overall health.

- **Hydration:** Proper hydration is essential for pain management, as dehydration can exacerbate discomfort.

- **Rest and Sleep:** Prioritizing adequate rest and quality sleep is crucial for pain management and physical recovery.

- **Holistic Modalities:** Explore alternative modalities like Reiki, energy healing, or reflexology,

which focus on balancing energy
and promoting holistic well-being.

Holistic approaches to physical well-being not only address immediate discomfort but also work to prevent future issues by promoting overall health and balance in the body. These practices empower individuals to take an active role in their physical well-being and enhance their overall quality of life.

CHAPTER 5

Emotional Well-Being

Emotional well-being is a vital component of holistic health, as it directly impacts physical, mental, and spiritual well-being.

5.1 Understanding Emotions in Holistic Health

Emotions are a fundamental aspect of holistic health, and understanding them is key to achieving overall well-being. Here are some key points to consider:

- **Emotional Intelligence:** Emotional intelligence involves recognizing, understanding, and effectively managing one's emotions. It also includes empathy for the emotions of others. Developing emotional intelligence is crucial for holistic health.

- **Emotion-Body Connection:** Emotions are not solely mental experiences; they have physical manifestations in the body. For example, stress can lead to muscle tension, while joy can result in a sense of lightness. Recognizing the mind-body connection is essential.

- **Emotional Triggers:** Identifying what triggers certain emotions is important for managing them effectively. This self-awareness can help individuals make healthier choices in response to emotional triggers.

- **Expression and Suppression:** Emotions need to be acknowledged and expressed rather than suppressed. Suppressed emotions can lead to physical and mental health issues over time.

- **Positive Emotions:** Cultivating positive emotions like gratitude, joy, and love can have a significant impact on overall well-being. These emotions can boost the immune system, reduce stress, and enhance mental clarity.

5.2 Stress Management Techniques

Stress is a common emotional challenge that can have a profound impact on holistic health. Managing stress effectively is crucial for overall well-being. Here are some stress management techniques to explore:

- **Mindfulness Meditation:** Mindfulness meditation involves focusing on the present moment without judgment. It can reduce stress, anxiety, and emotional reactivity.

- **Deep Breathing Exercises:** Practicing deep breathing techniques, such as diaphragmatic breathing or the 4-7-8 technique, can help activate the body's relaxation response.

- **Progressive Muscle Relaxation:** This technique involves systematically tensing and then relaxing different muscle groups in the body to reduce physical tension and stress.

- **Yoga:** Yoga combines physical postures, breath control, and meditation to promote relaxation and reduce stress.

- **Exercise:** Regular physical activity releases endorphins, which are natural mood elevators. Exercise can help manage stress and boost overall well-being.

- **Journaling:** Keeping a journal to express thoughts and emotions can be a helpful tool for self-reflection and stress relief.

- **Art and Creativity:** Engaging in creative activities like painting, drawing, or playing music can provide a therapeutic outlet for stress.

- **Time Management:** Effective time management techniques can reduce the stress associated with feeling overwhelmed or rushed.

- **Social Support:** Talking to friends, family, or a counselor can provide emotional support and perspective during stressful times.

5.3 Cultivating Emotional Resilience

Emotional resilience is the ability to bounce back from adversity and maintain mental and emotional well-being. Cultivating emotional resilience is a valuable skill in holistic health. Here's how to do it:

- **Self-Care:** Prioritize self-care practices that nurture your physical, mental, and emotional well-being. This includes getting enough sleep, eating well, and engaging in activities that bring you joy.

- **Positive Self-Talk:** Challenge negative self-talk and replace it with positive and constructive self-statements. Self-compassion is key to resilience.

- **Social Connections:** Maintain strong social connections and seek support from friends and loved ones when facing challenges.

- **Mindset Shifts:** Develop a growth mindset, which involves viewing challenges as opportunities for growth rather than insurmountable obstacles.

- **Coping Strategies:** Identify healthy coping strategies that work for you, such as seeking professional help, practicing relaxation techniques, or engaging in hobbies.

- **Emotional Regulation:** Learn techniques for regulating emotions, such as deep breathing, grounding exercises, and mindfulness practices.

- **Stress Reduction:** Continue to explore and practice stress management techniques to build resilience in the face of stressors.

- **Seeking Professional Help:** If needed, consider seeking the guidance of a therapist or counselor to work on emotional resilience and develop coping skills.

Emotional well-being is a dynamic aspect of holistic health that requires ongoing attention and self-awareness.

understanding emotions, managing stress effectively, and cultivating emotional resilience, individuals can navigate life's challenges with greater ease and maintain overall well-being.

CHAPTER 6

Holistic Approaches to Healing

Holistic approaches to healing encompass a wide range of alternative therapies and practices that address the physical, mental, emotional, and spiritual aspects of health.

6.1 Alternative Therapies and Their Benefits

Alternative therapies are non-conventional healing practices that focus on treating the whole person rather than just specific symptoms. They are often used alongside or as alternatives to traditional medical treatments. Here are some alternative therapies and their associated benefits:

1. **Acupuncture:** Acupuncture is an ancient Chinese practice that involves inserting thin needles into specific points on the body. It is believed to balance the body's energy flow (Qi) and can be used to alleviate pain, reduce stress, and promote overall well-being.

2. **Chiropractic Care:** Chiropractors use manual adjustments to the spine and joints to improve alignment and relieve musculoskeletal pain. Chiropractic care can be effective for managing back pain, headaches, and improving overall mobility.

3. **Homeopathy:** Homeopathy is based on the principle of "like

cures like." Tiny, highly diluted amounts of natural substances are used to stimulate the body's own healing mechanisms. It can be used for a wide range of conditions, including allergies, digestive issues, and emotional imbalances.

4. **Ayurveda:** Ayurveda is an ancient Indian system of medicine that emphasizes balance among the body, mind, and spirit. It utilizes diet, herbs, yoga, and meditation to promote health and prevent disease.

5. **Herbal Medicine:** Herbal medicine involves using plants and plant-based substances to treat various health conditions. Herbal remedies can support the body's natural healing processes and may be used for everything from

digestive disorders to sleep
disturbances.

6. **Energy Healing:** Energy healing
modalities like Reiki and Healing
Touch focus on balancing the
body's energy fields. They can
promote relaxation, reduce stress,
and support emotional and
physical healing.

7. **Massage Therapy:** Massage
therapy involves manipulating soft
tissues to promote relaxation,
relieve muscle tension, and
improve circulation. It can help
with pain management, stress
reduction, and overall well-being.

8. **Aromatherapy:** Aromatherapy
uses essential oils from plants to
promote physical and emotional
health. Different essential oils can
have various effects, such as

relaxation, energy enhancement, or
pain relief.

9. **Meditation and Mindfulness:**
    Meditation and mindfulness
    practices involve focused attention
    and awareness, helping individuals
    reduce stress, manage anxiety, and
    improve mental clarity. They can
    be used for both emotional and
    physical well-being.

10. **Biofeedback:** Biofeedback
    techniques provide individuals
    with real-time data about
    physiological processes such as
    heart rate, muscle tension, and skin
    temperature. This information
    helps individuals learn to control
    these functions and reduce stress
    and pain.

11. **Hypnotherapy:** Hypnotherapy
    uses guided relaxation and focused

attention to help individuals access
their subconscious mind. It can be
used to address a wide range of
issues, including phobias,
addiction, and chronic pain.

12. **Traditional Chinese Medicine
(TCM):** TCM includes practices
like herbal medicine, acupuncture,
cupping therapy, and tai chi. It
focuses on balancing the body's
vital energy (Qi) to promote health
and prevent disease.

13. **Naturopathy:** Naturopathic
doctors use a combination of
natural therapies, including
nutrition, herbal medicine, and
lifestyle counseling, to support
the body's natural healing
abilities.

Each of these alternative therapies
offers unique benefits in promoting

holistic health. They often prioritize the individual's well-being as a whole, working to address the root causes of health issues rather than just alleviating symptoms. When integrated into a holistic health approach, alternative therapies can complement conventional medicine and help individuals achieve greater overall well-being. It's essential to consult with qualified practitioners and healthcare providers when considering these therapies to ensure they are appropriate for your specific needs and health goals.

6.2 Holistic Health Modalities for Beginners

Holistic health modalities encompass various practices and therapies that promote well-being by addressing the interconnectedness of the mind, body, and spirit. Here are some modalities that are accessible and well-suited for beginners:

1. **Mindfulness Meditation:** Mindfulness meditation is a simple and highly accessible practice that involves paying focused attention to the present moment. Beginners can start with short sessions, gradually increasing the duration. Mindfulness can help reduce stress, enhance self-awareness, and improve overall mental well-being.

2. **Yoga:** Yoga is a holistic practice that combines physical postures (asanas), breath control (pranayama), and meditation. Many yoga classes cater to beginners, offering gentle and foundational poses to build

flexibility, strength, and mindfulness.

3. **Tai Chi:** Tai Chi is a gentle, flowing martial art that promotes balance, flexibility, and relaxation. Beginners can find beginner-friendly classes or online resources to start learning the basic movements.

4. **Aromatherapy:** Aromatherapy involves the use of essential oils to promote emotional and physical well-being. Beginners can explore different essential oils and learn how to use them safely through diffusion, topical application, or inhalation.

5. **Biofeedback:** Biofeedback is a non-invasive technique that helps individuals gain awareness and control over physiological

functions such as heart rate, muscle tension, and skin temperature. Many biofeedback devices and apps are beginner-friendly and offer guided sessions.

6. **Herbal Remedies:** Exploring herbal remedies can be a simple way to incorporate holistic health into daily life. Beginners can start with common herbs like chamomile for relaxation or ginger for digestion. It's important to research and use herbs safely.

7. **Journaling:** Keeping a journal can be a therapeutic practice for beginners. It allows individuals to express their thoughts, emotions, and experiences, leading to increased self-awareness and emotional processing.

8. **Breathing Exercises:** Deep breathing exercises are easy to learn and can have an immediate calming effect. Techniques like diaphragmatic breathing or the 4-7-8 method can be practiced anywhere and anytime.

9. **Crystal Healing:** Crystals are believed to have energetic properties that can influence well-being. Beginners can explore different crystals and their uses, such as amethyst for relaxation or rose quartz for self-love.

10. **Sound Healing:** Sound healing involves using specific sounds or frequencies, such as singing bowls or tuning forks, to promote relaxation and balance. Beginners can attend sound healing sessions or explore sound healing recordings.

11. **Guided Imagery:** Guided imagery involves using mental images to promote relaxation and reduce stress. There are many guided imagery apps and recordings designed for beginners.

12. **Progressive Muscle Relaxation:** This relaxation technique involves systematically tensing and then relaxing different muscle groups in the body. It can help beginners release physical tension and promote relaxation.

13. **Holistic Nutrition:** Beginners can start by incorporating more whole foods, fruits, and vegetables into their diet. Learning about the nutritional benefits of different foods can be a valuable step toward holistic nutrition.

14. **Mandala Coloring:** Coloring mandalas is a relaxing and creative practice that can promote mindfulness and stress reduction. Beginners can find mandala coloring books or printable designs online.

15. **Walking in Nature:** Connecting with nature is a holistic practice that's readily accessible. Taking leisurely walks in natural settings can reduce stress, boost mood, and enhance overall well-being.

it's essential to explore these modalities at your own pace and find what resonates with you. Consider seeking guidance or classes from experienced practitioners, when possible, as they can provide valuable insights and support your holistic health journey. Remember that consistency and patience are key as you integrate these practices into your daily life.

6.3 Combining Conventional and Holistic Approaches

1. **Open Communication:** Effective integration begins with open and honest communication between you and your healthcare providers. Inform your conventional healthcare provider about any holistic therapies or practices you are considering, and discuss any potential interactions or concerns.

2. **Collaborative Care:** Seek healthcare providers who are open to integrative approaches and willing to work collaboratively. Integrative or functional medicine

practitioners are often well-versed in combining conventional and holistic therapies.

3. **Comprehensive Assessment:** Conventional medicine is valuable for diagnosing and managing acute and severe conditions. Holistic approaches can complement this by addressing underlying causes, promoting prevention, and managing chronic conditions.

4. **Personalized Treatment Plans:** Work with healthcare providers to develop personalized treatment plans that incorporate both conventional and holistic therapies. These plans should consider your unique health goals, preferences, and any contraindications.

5. **Informed Decision-Making:** Make informed decisions about your healthcare. Research and educate yourself about both conventional and holistic therapies, including their potential benefits and risks.

6. **Evidence-Based Holistic Practices:** Choose holistic practices that have a strong evidence base and are supported by scientific research. This ensures that you are incorporating effective and safe therapies into your regimen.

7. **Mindful Medication Use:** If you are taking medications prescribed by a conventional healthcare provider, inform them of any supplements or herbal remedies you are considering. Some

interactions between medications
and supplements can occur.

8. **Holistic Lifestyle:** Embrace a
holistic lifestyle that includes
balanced nutrition, regular
physical activity, stress
management, and healthy sleep
patterns. These foundational
aspects of well-being are
compatible with both conventional
and holistic approaches.

9. **Gradual Integration:** Start by
integrating one or a few holistic
practices into your routine and
gradually expand as you become
more comfortable and informed.
Small changes can have a
significant impact over time.

10. **Monitoring Progress:** Regularly
assess and monitor your progress.
Keep track of how conventional

and holistic approaches are affecting your health and well-being, and adjust your approach as needed.

11. **Holistic Practitioners:** Seek guidance from qualified holistic practitioners, such as naturopathic doctors, registered dietitians, or licensed acupuncturists. These professionals can provide expert advice and help you navigate holistic therapies safely.

12. **Preventive Focus:** Holistic approaches often emphasize prevention. Use these practices to maintain overall health and prevent illness, complementing the reactive nature of conventional medicine.

13. **Holistic Therapies for Well-Being:** Holistic therapies like

mindfulness, yoga, and relaxation techniques can enhance your emotional and mental well-being. These practices are valuable additions to conventional mental health treatments.

14. **Patient Empowerment:** Taking an active role in your healthcare is essential. Understand that you have the right to make informed choices about your well-being, and advocate for your holistic health goals with your healthcare providers.

15. **Holistic Support Groups:** Joining support groups or communities focused on holistic health can provide valuable resources, guidance, and shared experiences.

The goal of combining conventional and holistic approaches is to enhance your overall well-being, improve your quality of life, and achieve optimal health outcomes. It's important to work closely with healthcare providers who respect your choices and support your holistic health journey. This integrated approach allows you to leverage the strengths of both paradigms and address your health needs comprehensively.

CHAPTER 7

Holistic Lifestyle Habits

A holistic lifestyle is centered around the concept of balance and harmony among the physical, mental, emotional, and spiritual aspects of well-being.

7.1 Creating a Holistic Daily Routine

A well-structured daily routine can serve as a foundation for a holistic lifestyle, promoting overall well-being. Here are steps to create a holistic daily routine:

1. Start with Morning Rituals:

- **Morning Meditation or Mindfulness:** Begin your day with a short meditation or mindfulness practice to set a positive tone and clear your mind.

- **Gratitude Journaling:** Write down a few things you're grateful for each morning to foster a positive mindset.

2. Balanced Nutrition:

- **Mindful Breakfast:** Enjoy a balanced breakfast that includes whole grains, fruits or vegetables, and a source of protein to provide sustained energy throughout the morning.

- **Hydration:** Start your day with a glass of water to rehydrate your body after sleep.

3. Movement and Exercise:

- **Physical Activity:** Incorporate some form of physical activity into your morning routine, whether it's yoga, stretching, a brisk walk, or a workout session.

4. Mindful Work or Productivity:

- **Work or Study:** Dedicate focused time to your work or study tasks, incorporating short breaks for relaxation and movement.

- **Mindful Work Habits:** Practice mindfulness during work, which can enhance productivity and reduce stress.

5. Nutrient-Dense Meals:

- **Lunch:** Choose a balanced, nutrient-dense lunch to maintain energy levels throughout the day.

6. Mindful Breaks:

- **Midday Break:** Take a short break to practice deep breathing, stretch, or simply relax for a few minutes.

- **Mindful Eating:** Pay attention to your lunch, savoring each bite and eating without distractions.

7. Afternoon Rejuvenation:

- **Mindful Movement:** Incorporate mindful movement or exercise in the afternoon to boost energy and reduce stress.

- **Healthy Snack:** If needed, enjoy a healthy snack to maintain stable blood sugar levels.

8. Evening Wind-Down:

- **Mindful Dinner:** Eat a light, balanced dinner that is easily digestible.

- **Evening Walk:** Take a leisurely walk to unwind and reflect on your day.

9. Relaxation and Reflection:

- **Evening Meditation:** Engage in a calming meditation or relaxation practice before bedtime.

- **Journaling:** Reflect on your day, jotting down any insights, challenges, or positive experiences.

10. Prioritize Sleep:

- **Quality Sleep:** Aim for at least 7-9 hours of restful sleep each night. Create a calming bedtime routine and maintain a consistent sleep schedule.

11. Digital Detox:

- **Screen-Free Time:** Allocate time in the evening for a digital detox. Avoid screens at least an hour before bedtime to promote better sleep.

12. Self-Care:

- **Regular Self-Care:** Schedule regular self-care practices, such as a weekly bath, reading a book, or enjoying a hobby you love.

13. Mindful Connection:

- **Quality Time with Loved Ones:** Spend quality time with friends and family, nurturing social connections and emotional well-being.

14. Reflect and Adjust:

- **Daily Review:** Before bedtime, reflect on your day and evaluate how well you adhered to your holistic routine. Make adjustments as needed.

Creating a holistic daily routine is about fostering balance, self-care, and mindful living. Customize your routine to align with your personal preferences and needs, and remember that consistency is key to experiencing the full benefits of a holistic lifestyle. Over time, these daily habits can promote physical health, mental clarity, emotional well-being, and a deeper sense of connection with yourself and the world around you.

7.2 Sleep, Rest, and Recovery

Sleep, rest, and recovery are essential components of a holistic lifestyle. They play a crucial role in overall well-being, affecting physical, mental, and emotional health. Here are some key considerations for incorporating quality sleep, rest, and recovery into your holistic lifestyle:

1. Prioritize Quality Sleep:

- **Consistent Schedule:** Maintain a consistent sleep schedule by going to bed and waking up at the same times each day, even on weekends.

- **Create a Relaxing Bedtime Routine:** Wind down before bedtime with calming activities such as reading, gentle stretching, or meditation. Avoid stimulating activities and screens at least an hour before sleep.

- **Comfortable Sleep Environment:** Ensure your bedroom is conducive to sleep. This includes a comfortable mattress and pillows, adequate room temperature, and minimal noise and light.

- **Limit Caffeine and Alcohol:** Avoid caffeine and alcohol close to bedtime, as they can disrupt sleep patterns.

- **Mindful Eating:** Finish eating at least a few hours before bedtime to allow for proper digestion.

- **Stress Management:** Practice relaxation techniques to manage stress and anxiety, which can interfere with sleep. Mindfulness meditation and deep breathing exercises can be particularly helpful.

2. Rest and Recovery:

- **Scheduled Breaks:** Incorporate regular breaks during the day, especially if you have a busy schedule. Short breaks for relaxation, stretching, or deep breathing can boost energy and reduce stress.

- **Power Naps:** Short power naps (around 20-30 minutes) can provide a quick energy boost during the day, but avoid long naps that can disrupt nighttime sleep.

- **Active Recovery:** After intense physical activity or workouts, engage in active recovery activities such as gentle yoga, swimming, or walking to aid muscle recovery and reduce post-exercise soreness.

- **Massage and Bodywork:** Consider occasional massages or bodywork sessions to relax muscles, improve circulation, and promote overall physical and mental relaxation.

3. Listen to Your Body:

- Pay attention to your body's signals for rest and recovery. If you feel fatigued or mentally drained, prioritize rest.

- Avoid overloading your schedule with commitments or tasks that leave you with minimal downtime.

- Practice self-compassion and allow yourself to rest without guilt when needed.

4. Mindful Rest:

- Engage in mindful rest, which involves consciously relaxing and fully immersing yourself in the present moment. This can be done through meditation, nature walks, or simply sitting quietly.

- Avoid overstimulating activities, especially before bedtime, to facilitate a more restful state of mind.

5. Technology Detox:

- Implement technology detox periods during the day, especially in the evening. Reduce screen time and avoid electronic devices at least an hour before bedtime to improve sleep quality.

6. Balance Work and Leisure:

- Strive for a balanced lifestyle that includes both work and leisure activities. Avoid overworking or overcommitting to responsibilities at the expense of rest and relaxation.

7. Holistic Practices:

- Incorporate holistic practices like meditation, yoga, and deep breathing into your daily routine. These activities promote relaxation and mental clarity, enhancing overall well-being.

8. Seek Professional Help:

- If you struggle with sleep disorders, chronic fatigue, or high levels of stress, consider seeking professional help. A healthcare provider or therapist can provide guidance and support tailored to your needs.

Quality sleep and effective rest and recovery practices are foundational for maintaining physical health, mental clarity, and emotional resilience. By prioritizing these aspects of a holistic lifestyle, you can optimize your well-being and enhance your ability to cope with life's challenges. Remember that the key is to find a balance that works for you and to listen to your body's signals for rest and restoration.

CHAPTER 8

Putting It All Together

8.1 Developing Your Holistic Health Plan

Creating a holistic health plan is the culmination of your journey towards overall well-being. Here's how to develop your personalized plan:

- **Assessment:** Begin by assessing your current physical, mental, emotional, and spiritual health. Identify areas that need improvement and set clear goals.

- **Goals:** Define specific, measurable, achievable, relevant, and time-bound (SMART) goals for each aspect of your holistic health. For example, your goals might include improving nutrition, managing stress, or enhancing relationships.

- **Prioritization:** Prioritize your goals based on their importance and urgency. Focus on one or two key areas at a time to avoid feeling overwhelmed.

- **Action Steps:** Break down each goal into actionable steps. Create a list of activities, practices, and changes you need to implement to achieve your goals.

- **Timeline:** Set a realistic timeline for achieving each goal. Be flexible and adjust as needed, understanding that holistic health is an ongoing journey.

- **Resources:** Identify the resources and support you need to succeed. This may include seeking guidance from healthcare providers, enlisting the support of friends and family, or accessing educational materials.

- **Holistic Practices:** Incorporate holistic practices into your daily routine, aligning them with your goals. For example, if stress reduction is a goal, prioritize daily meditation or yoga sessions.

- **Review and Adapt:** Regularly review your holistic health plan, tracking your progress and making adjustments as needed. Celebrate your achievements along the way.

8.2 Tracking Your Progress

Tracking your progress is essential for staying accountable and making necessary adjustments. Here are some tips for effective progress tracking:

- **Journaling:** Maintain a holistic health journal to record your experiences, thoughts, and feelings. Track your daily practices, challenges, and successes.

- **Measuring Metrics:** For physical health goals, track relevant metrics such as weight, blood pressure, or fitness levels. For mental and emotional goals, note changes in mood, stress levels, or sleep quality.

- **Visual Aids:** Create visual aids, such as charts or graphs, to visualize your progress over time. This can provide motivation and clarity.

- **Accountability Partner:** Share your holistic health plan with a trusted friend or family member who can serve as an accountability partner. Regular check-ins can help you stay on track.

- **Use Technology:** There are many apps and digital tools available for tracking various aspects of your holistic health, from nutrition and exercise to meditation and sleep.

8.3 Embracing a Holistic Lifestyle

Embracing a holistic lifestyle is a continuous journey that involves integrating all aspects of your well-being into daily life. Here's how to fully embrace a holistic lifestyle:

- **Mindfulness:** Practice mindfulness in all aspects of your life. Be present in the moment, whether you're eating, exercising, working, or spending time with loved ones.

- **Self-Care:** Prioritize self-care as an essential part of your routine. Regularly engage in activities that nourish your body, mind, and spirit.

- **Balance:** Strive for balance in all areas of your life, including work, relationships, and leisure. Avoid extremes and prioritize moderation.

- **Flexibility:** Be flexible and adaptable. Understand that setbacks and challenges are a natural part of life. Approach them with resilience and a growth mindset.

- **Connection:** Nurture your connections with others and with nature. Recognize the interconnectedness of all living things and the importance of fostering a sense of community.

- **Continuous Learning:** Commit to lifelong learning and personal growth. Stay open to new ideas, practices, and experiences that contribute to your holistic well-being.

- **Gratitude:** Cultivate a sense of gratitude for the blessings in your life. Regularly express appreciation for the people, experiences, and opportunities that enrich your journey.

- **Joy:** Prioritize joy and happiness as fundamental aspects of your holistic lifestyle. Engage in activities and practices that bring you genuine joy and fulfillment.

embracing a holistic lifestyle is a personal and evolving process. It's about aligning your choices and actions with your values, goals, and the principles of holistic health. By doing so, you can experience a profound transformation in your overall well-being, achieving a state of balance, harmony, and vitality that encompasses all aspects of your life.

www.ingramcontent.com/pod-product-compliance
Lightning Source LLC
Chambersburg PA
CBHW070839260726
48660CB00005B/2086